The HCG Diet Bible

The Essential Guide to the Popular HCG Diet Plan

M. Smith

The HCG Diet Bible

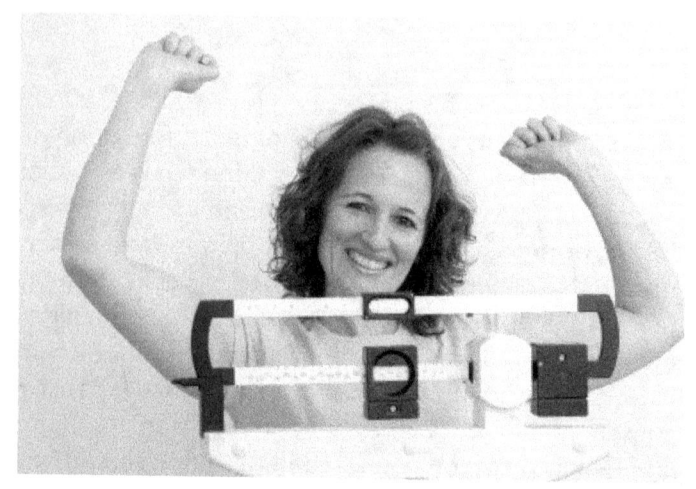

HCG Diet Success

Table of Contents

"You must begin to think of yourself as becoming the person you want to be".
David Viscott

The HCG Diet Bible

A Review of the HCG Diet Plan

If you have a serious weight problem and are searching for a diet plan that offers quick and long term results, the HCG Diet Plan may be what you're looking for. The HCG (Human Chorionic Gonadotropin) Diet Plan is an incredible method to get rid of unwanted pounds and, you'll keep them off because it also restores a sluggish metabolism.

HCG is a hormone found in cells that make up the placenta in a pregnant woman as early as eleven days after conception. After 11 days, the HCG hormone can also be found in a pregnant woman's urine. This hormone has the important job of providing nutrients to the fetus, helping it grow into a healthy baby.

Author and outspoken advocate of holistic methods for weight loss, Kevin Trudeau, introduced the concept of the HCG Diet in his highly touted book, "The Weight Loss Cure," citing the findings based on research of the late British doctor, A.T.W. Simeons. Dr. Simeons dedicated many years to studying weight loss brought about by injections of HCG, and his success with the plan spanned a period of over 50 years.

The HCG Diet works on the premise of "resetting" the hypothalamus gland – a gland that helps the neurotransmitters in the brain to receive messages correctly. These neurotransmitters are necessary for the functioning of the brain's most potent hormones – Nor epinephrine, Serotonin, Acetylcholine and Dopamine – which, in turn, affect the imbalances in our bodies.

Some crucial imbalances that can prevent weight loss when the hypothalamus gland isn't working properly are metabolism, hunger, salt cravings and energy levels. There is also an important link of the hypothalamus to the organization of our mood levels. A certain type of mood could make us ravenously hungry so that we reach for every food in sight just to stop the cravings that our brain is making us think is real.

Injections or oral consumption of the HCG hormone regulates and resets the hypothalamus gland so that it's working for you rather than against you in weight loss realizations. Injections can be performed by your doctor easily and quickly, while oral alternatives are becoming more available, thanks to Dr. Daniel Beluccio, who created the protocol.

Both Simeon and Trudeau advocate a regimen of herbal teas such as wu, green tea and chamomile while embarking on the HCG Diet Plan and Trudeau additionally recommends supplements and cleansing methods for eliminating toxins in the body.

This amazing HCG Diet Plan actually achieves fast and permanent weight loss, reshaping the body as the pounds melt off. It's inexpensive and works for both men and women in helping each attain sought after weight loss goals.

Do HCG Diets Really Work?

The answer to the title question is, "yes" – but only if you stick to it – and that's true for any weight loss plan. Thousands have stuck to HCG Diets and lost a remarkable amount of weight and inches. This incredible plan has been around since 1954, but has only received an outpouring of recognition when author and weight loss guru, Kevin Trudeau, published his book, "The Weight Loss Cure."

In "The Weight Loss Cure," Trudeau chronicles the research and findings of the late Dr. A.T.W Simeon, who made remarkable breakthroughs in weight loss of obese patients. For years, Dr. Simeon injected patients with a glycoprotein hormone called HCG (Human Chorionic Gonadotropin), a hormone only produced during women's pregnancies – and produced dramatic results.

A low calorie diet (500 calories per day) is also an essential part in the beginning of HCG Diets because it helps to rid your body of abnormal fat and begin the transformation of your body image. Following an HCG Diet plan also regulates a listless metabolism, which is necessary for your body to effectively burn off future calories.

Obesity is becoming a serious problem in today's society, and HCG Diets may hold the solution to our future health. Obesity is a big part of the reason for health problems such as diabetes, heart attacks and strokes, not to mention low-self-esteem and poor self-image. The fact that those who partake in HCG Diets tend to keep the weight off is an extra benefit.

Weight loss is now one of the most money-making pursuits today. People everywhere are joining weight loss clubs, drinking and eating diet drinks and foods and purchasing fitness equipment in an attempt to lose calories and get in shape.

HCG Diets are relatively inexpensive and there are no special foods, fads, pills or any other form of weight loss treatment that you need to adhere to. The HCG hormone is usually injected by a physician, but oral treatments are becoming more popular.

Before Kevin Trudeau included HCG Diets in his book, he utilized the treatment for himself – losing 45 pounds in six weeks. In an infomercial, he touted that no exercise was needed to achieve the weight loss and that his energy level soared while his eating habits drastically changed for the better.

There's an added benefit for HCG Diets that isn't as well documented as the weight loss factor – youth. The HCG hormone injections have the extra advantage of bringing the glow of youth back to your appearance.

If you've always failed when trying to lose those unwanted pounds, research the HCG Diets and talk to your health care provider about whether this plan may work best for you.

HCG Diet Dangers – Truth or Fiction?

There may be danger to just about anything you do that changes your body's chemistry. That's why it's important that you check with your health care provider before taking any new drugs or undertaking a strenuous exercise program or unusual diet plan. You may have heard about the HCG diet plan and wonder if there are any HCG diet dangers or side effects that you should be aware of.

The HCG (human Chorionic Gonadotrophin) injections and diet plan has been bombarded with bad and inaccurate information that's simply not true. But, there are some parts of the diet plan that could be bad for you – just as other diet plans may harm you if you have certain health conditions.

Information about HCG diet dangers can be provided by people who are misinformed or are trying to convince you that their diet plan is better. That's why it's imperative that you do your own research and be informed of the true facts about the HCG hormone and diet plan. Then, you can make an informed decision about whether or not the plan is right for you.

HCG hormone injections might present a problem if you don't know what you're doing. Fortunately, there are now oral drops that you can take sublingually and will provide the same effectiveness if you're trying to lose weight.

You don't need a prescription to purchase the drops. Online sites offer information and products that can be delivered to you at your home. Just be sure you know who you're buying the product from. As with any weight loss program, there are scams out there.

The HCG diet plan is easy to follow. Many who have followed the plan have reported that hunger and cravings were eradicated because of the effectiveness of the injections or drops. These dieters also reported that they had more energy to exercise and that the pounds virtually melted off.

HCG diet dangers are lessened because the diet is done in stages rather than all at once and shocking your system. The first stage is a detoxifying stage, where you drink lots of water per day and exercise can be a simple morning walk. After your body and mind are detoxified, you're fully prepared for the next stage.

The second phase of the HCG diet involves ingesting large amounts of calories. This is designed to restart your metabolism so that fat can be burned efficiently and quickly. During this two-day period, you can eat whatever you want.

The third, and actual diet phase, involves eating only 500 calories per day as you're taking HCG hormone injections or drops. Again, HCG drops are recommended over the injections if you're not familiar with giving them. HCG diet dangers can be eliminated by checking with your doctor first to make sure it doesn't interfere with a medical condition or other drugs you may be taking.

HCG Drops - Magic or Miracle?

People are asking questions about HCG (human Chorionic Gonadotropin) Drops – are they magical and do they perform a miracle for those desperate to lose weight? Actually, HCG Drops are a scientific breakthrough comprised of a special hormone that melts away fat cells when activated. The HCG hormone lies in the body's molecular structure and has been touted as the "fat burning hormone."

Claims of weight loss from individuals during a 30 day time period range from15 to 25 pounds. Users of HCG Drops also claim to have unbridled energy and improved body shape – without exercising. There are no pre-packaged foods to purchase and no weight-loss meetings to attend.

HCG Drops isn't based on a fad diet program that makes you purchase name-brand products and spend numerous, excruciating hours in a fitness center. The only thing you have to do in the beginning is eat fewer calories. But, no specific foods are recommended – and when HCG Drops begin to activate, you can eat as you normally would.

People who have used HCG Drops claim that their appetites are drastically reduced and energy levels are improved. Weight loss is rapid on the HCG Drops plan, and that spurs you on to continue. The HCG hormone stimulates the hypothalamus gland, which regulates your metabolism – and when your metabolism is working properly, you'll achieve the proper weight.

Best of all, the weight won't pile back on after you reach your desired goal. Once your body becomes balanced inside, you'll lose the cravings or desires to eat more than you need to maintain the perfect weight for your body.

Most fad diets and exercise regimes aren't realistic in today's world. Starvation diets eventually become more than our minds and bodies can endure and we starve ourselves for weeks or months before binge eating to satisfy our cravings. The HCG Drops are based on scientific research and evidence of success since 1954.

Research of the HCG hormone was done by Dr. A.T.W. Simeon and turned studies for weight loss around when Kevin Trudeau published Simeon's results and the theory behind the hormone in his book, "The Weight Loss Cure." Since then, the buzz about HCG Drops has risen to a crescendo that's difficult to ignore.

Do your own research about HCG Drops and discover whether this may be the answer you've searched for to completely and finally get rid of your weight loss problem. You'll find a plethora of information about HCG Drops on the Internet, and some books (such as Trudeau's "The Weight Loss Cure) that explains the HCG Drops in more detail.

HCG Drops aren't snake oil magic – nor is it a miracle. Its premise is based on scientific evidence and is readily available for anyone who has a weight problem. It's best to consult with your health care provider before engaging in any weight loss plan.

HCG for Weight Loss Is Quick and Effective

Are you tired of trying diet after diet, joining fitness center or spending tons of money on equipment and pre-packaged meals that leave you gagging? Using HCG (human Chorionic Gonadotropin) for weight loss has been proven to be safe, work quickly and even give you a new lease on life.

HCG for weight loss fits into the category of natural remedies for losing weight safely. The HCG hormone is an important chemical that's naturally produced by the placenta in pregnant women to help bring nutrients to the fetus. When used as a weight loss option, the HCG hormone effectively stimulates the hypothalamus gland, which regulates metabolism and other triggers that promote weight loss.

The theory behind stimulating the hypothalamus gland in pregnant women is that while they're "eating for two," they need extra nutrients for both themselves and the babies they're carrying. They'll also gain extra energy from the process. But, when the hypothalamus is stimulated in males or non-pregnant women, the result is that fat gets burned twice as fast and effectively – even without exercise.

Also, the HCG hormone is one that is found in every man and woman – but remains dormant in body cells. The synthetic HCG hormone, which is used for weight loss purposes is now approved b the FDA and produces the same benefits as the natural hormone found in pregnant women.

There are two ways to enjoy the benefits of HCG for weight loss. One is through injections given by your doctor, and the other is to use HCG drops by releasing them under your tongue before meals. The HCG hormone will do the work of stimulating the hypothalamus gland and the fat will begin to disappear.

One of the best advantages of HCG for weight loss is that you'll begin to see results almost immediately. In Kevin Trudeau's blockbuster book, "The Weight Loss Cure," he chronicles his own weight loss while taking the HCG hormone and the results are startling.

Trudeau's weight loss journey is detailed in the book, and he inserts "before and after" photos so that you can actually see the results. Other testimonials for the use of HCG for weight loss include many diabetics who claim that their lives were changed for the better after losing weight and balancing the chemicals in their bodies.

Other satisfied consumers of the HCG hormone have said that they have a new lease on life and more energy than they ever thought possible. Some say that it was the easiest way to lose weight and keep it off that they've ever experienced, even though at the beginning of the diet, the calories are highly restrictive – only 500 calories per day.

If you're looking for a diet plan to end obesity once and for all, research the HCG for weight loss plan yourself and decide if this method might work for you.

HCG Injections Risks and Rewards

If you're serious about losing weight and have tried every diet plan known to man, you may be considering using HCG injections. You may also want to know what the risks and rewards of this highly touted and effective weight loss method before you begin.

HCG (Human Chorionic Gonadotropin) injections are fairly expensive – especially when performed by a health care provider. Many people give themselves the injections, but that should only be done if you're confident in the procedure. HCG injection "kits" are available online and can be purchased in increments, so you're not out a ton of money all at once.

Unless you know what you're doing, injecting yourself can cause bruising and soreness. You might also develop a cyst, even though the chances of that are slim. Fortunately, if you don't know how to give injections, an oral form of HCG is available and it's said to produce the same results.

hCC is a hormone produced by the placenta during pregnancy to provide the fetus and the mother with the nutrients they must have. A synthetic form of HCG, however, has been proven to help people achieve weight loss at an incredible rate when combined with the HCG diet plan. Studies show that hGC injections work because it resets the metabolism to burn unwanted fat.

Could HCG injections be the miracle weight loss method that everyone has been searching and hoping for? Kevin Trudeau, controversial author of "The Weight Loss

Cure," tried HCG injections on himself and produced startling results which are touted in his book.

One of the best things that Trudeau found about HCG injections that even though it should be combined with a low calorie diet for a few weeks – he wasn't hungry during the time he was taking the injections. The HCG hormone also has the effect of changing important brain receptors that tell us when we're hungry, and taking the HCG injections stopped the hunger pains.

After the metabolism has been reset, it keeps working correctly, even after you stop taking the HCG injections. And, it's not a fly-by-night or fad diet plan. The late doctor, A.T.W. Simeon, researched the effects of HCG injections over 30 years ago. When Trudeau came across the studies, he decided to do some research of his own and that's when he revealed the HCG hormone injections as a weight loss breakthrough.

Trudeau brought the HCG weight loss plan to millions with his book and now people are flocking online and to their health care provider to find out more about this "miraculous" weight loss cure. In fact, the diet plan has become so popular that researchers found a way to produce a sublingual oral produce since the injection method scared many people away.

HCG injections can be the weight loss tool that helps you finally lose the pounds you may have been trying to get rid of your entire life. A steady supply of the synthetic hormone is required for up to 45 days in order to reap the full benefits. Decide for yourself if the reward of a leaner you outweighs the risks.

How HCG Hormones Help You Lose Weight

Your first thought when you heard about HCG Hormones might have been, "How can a hormone that helps a pregnant woman and her fetus receive nutrients help me lose weight?" Actually, it makes perfect sense when you read on and find out about how HCG hormones interact with your body and the HCG diet plan.

It's true that HCG (human Chorionic Gonadotropin) hormones are necessary for pregnant women and are produced by the cells in the placenta to ensure healthy fetus development. The rest of us also have HCG hormones in our cells, but they've been removed from our bodies, possibly by chemicals contained in certain foods.

If you've ever had a need to take antibiotics, the balance of the digestive system could be affected, causing you to lose the valuable HCG hormones. HCG loss could occur because of a Candida yeast overgrowth caused by the chemical imbalance in the digestive system.

Having no HCG in your system means that the hypothalamus gland is affected. This gland controls body fat and emotions that might trigger overeating and also helps form the reproductive glands during the puberty stage. When synthetic HCG hormones are added to the system by injections or oral drops, they allow fat to be extracted from cells in which they're stored.

After the fat is removed, the cells become expendable, so the body breaks them down and absorbs them into the system. The body may then replace the cells with water (water retention) and since water weighs more than fat, you may even register heavier on the scale for a short while. When you're on the 500 calories per day HCG diet, water is often retained to make up for the rapid loss of fat cells.

If you're following the HCG diet plan and taking HCG hormones, you'll eventually rid your body of the water weight gain through the urine – and, it may seem like you're making a beeline for the bathroom most of the day and night for awhile. What follows will be a notable weight loss on the scale.

Eventually – after a few days – the weight loss decreases from day to day after the initial large amount of weight loss when the water is released from the body. Men can sometimes pull off a larger amount of weight loss than women despite the fact that they're following the diet explicitly. The reason for that is the different ways in which men and women retain water.

Religiously taking HCG hormones in either injection or oral drop form and following the prescribed diet plan should help you lose up to 30 pounds in a month. Some dieters lose less and some more – but this remarkable plan can end your weight woes forever – without having to purchase special foods or enter into a strenuous exercise regime.

HCG hormones can definitely help you lose weight and develop a new lease on life because the weight loss usually stays off after the metabolism is reset.

How to Raise Your HCG Level

Human Chorionic Gonadotrophin (HCG) is a hormone manufactured by the placenta in pregnant women. The reason why women produce HCG has to do with providing necessary nutrients for both the woman and the fetus. In pregnant women, the HCG level usually doubles every few hours of her pregnancy. If a woman has low levels of HCG in her blood, that usually indicates a problem, such as an imminent miscarriage.

When a physician sees a low HCG level in an expectant mother, he or she may recommend certain methods to increase the level, even though that's no guarantee for a healthy pregnancy. If nothing is done or the physician finds no HCG in the pregnant woman, the lining of the uterus begins to deteriorate and the woman will begin her menstrual cycle.

To increase the HCG level, a doctor may recommend avoiding diuretics such as caffeine before being given the HCG test because diuretics decrease the amount of HCG in the sample by moving it more rapidly through the system. Recommendations may also include synthetic HCG injections, which is a common procedure during fertility treatments.

A recent weight loss phenomenon is based on the premise that increasing the HCG level of obese people stimulates the hypothalamus gland and resets the metabolism, thus burning fat quickly and more effectively.

Increasing the HCG level for weight loss purposes is said to be safe for both women and men and is a natural hormone, found in all humans. In non-pregnant humans, the hormone is found in body cells and is often dormant until stimulated. Those who have used HCG hormone drops or injections reported that their hunger levels were reduced and they had an abundant supply of energy while taking them.

For others, who are desperately trying to lose weight and have tried every diet, exercise program, homeopathic remedies and any other remedy that's supposed to help drop unwanted pounds, this may be the answer to all their diet needs. People who have experience weight loss from the HCG hormone say that they did not put the weight back on after finishing the program designed to increase the HCG level.

One side effect that has been reported by young women who have increased their HCG level by taking the synthetic injections or drops is that it affects their fertility and some experience irregular menstrual cycles. If you're a young woman with fertility problems, you should definitely try the HCG hormone under a doctor's care.

HCG supplements come in the form of injections and sublingual drops that can be inserted under the tongue. The FDA has recently approved HCG and now, anyone can purchase the synthetic hormone either online or from a health care provider or pharmaceutical company.

Tasty HCG Recipes Can Enhance the HCG Diet Plan

Have you read about the HCG diet plan and wonder how in the world you can survive the second phase which limits your caloric intake to 500 calories per day? If so, take note of the tasty recipes found online on HCG websites – some concocted by Dr. Simeon (creator of the HCG diet plan) himself.

Not only does the HCG diet plan work, but you don't have to deprive yourself. There are recipes available that are carefully designed to give you the nutrients you need while aiding the HCG hormone you're taking by injection or oral drops. Just any old diet won't work – the HCG diet plan only works at the optimal level when you're following the tried and true path of the diet.

The HCG recipes include a yummy Cream of Asparagus Soup, cleverly put together with cottage cheese rather than cream, generous portions of asparagus, seasoned with onion, parsley, basil, salt and pepper. You can even enjoy a bowl of soup with a breadstick!

Crock Pot Beef Chili is another tasty entrée recipe and a Strawberry or Chocolate Smoothie can wake you up in the morning or help soothe you to sleep at night. Your taste buds will be titillated by the Orange Asian Chicken and you'll wonder how you ever lived without the Strawberry Chicken Salad.

By enjoying the HCG recipes that are offered online and in many books about the HCG diet, you shouldn't have a problem - even during the restricted, 500 calorie phase of the diet. But, before you improvise a recipe, be sure that it's allowed on the diet. For example, if the recipe calls for chicken breast, don't improvise by using turkey or beef – it won't work as well.

Basically, the HCG diet consists of lean meat, fresh fruits and vegetables, but we can do so much more today to make the HCG recipes palatable. Seasonings and helpful additions to the recipes enhance the flavors and make it simple and enjoyable to stay on the diet plan – especially knowing that the results are going to be phenomenal.

Adhering to the diet while taking HCG hormone injections or oral drops maximizes the result of what the HCG hormone is doing for your body. The food that your body is receiving during the diet phase is being used to fuel your energy level while the hormone is breaking down the unwanted fat cells in the body.

The result of that formula means that you'll be burning up to 4,000 calories per day of stored fat and losing 1 or 2 pounds per day. This may seem unbelievable, but when you understand how the HCG hormone works in connection with your body, it makes perfect sense.

This amazing synthetic hormone actually resets your metabolism by triggering the hypothalamus to bring stored fat into the bloodstream. It protects and keeps your muscle mass and good fat while ridding your body of the toxins that make you miserable.

The hormone, combined with a diet full of tasty HCG recipes, might be the answer to getting rid of unwanted weight – and keeping it off.

The Best Places to Buy HCG

If you're searching for places to buy HCG injections or oral drops, you've done all the preliminary research and realize that it's the diet plan you need to once and for all lose unwanted pounds. You also know that you shouldn't buy HCG from any old distributor. You should find one with a good reputation and that you can count on to provide you with information you'll need about the diet.

Online sources are great places from which to purchase everything you'll need for your HCG diet plan. If you plan to follow Dr. Simeon's protocol, then you'll want injectable HCG, but if giving yourself daily injections sounds intimidating, you may want to find a place to buy HCG in its oral form.

Some states restrict injectable needles to those with prescriptions, such as insulin for diabetics. But, the oral form is easy to find both online and in some health pharmacies, so you shouldn't have any trouble.

Sites such as the HCG Weight Loss Search provide customized Google searches so that the actual search is streamlined to give you information about your specific search – such as HCG diet plan. It's best to choose U.S.A. companies to provide your HCG supplies rather than foreign suppliers because the ingredients are better regulated before sale.

There are providers who claim to offer pure HCG synthetic hormone injections and drops, but the actual product contains other ingredients. During your research, you should look for HCG that is processed at a "federally registered pharmaceutical laboratory in compliance with FDA regulations governing pharmaceutical manufacturing facilities."

This official document that contains the guidelines for homeopathic manufacturing practices in the United States was put together by the Homeopathic Pharmacopoeia of the United States and products from these laboratories are strictly regulated.

There are scams in everything though, so finding the right source for the HCG hormone is extremely important to your health and safety – and for the integrity of the product. You should know that a recent scam involving HCG supply websites have popped up. These fraudulent sites require Western Union or bank transfers to complete a transaction.

If you have a concern about a company's reputation, contact Paypal, MasterCard or Visa to be sure you're protected against this type of fraud. And, never send money by Western Union or bank transfer unless you've thoroughly checked out the company and have received recommendations from other HCG dieters.

When you're researching a site from which to buy HCG products, find out if the online site is updated regularly. Some also provide reviews about the quality of the product and the ease of use of the site and post ongoing blogs from customers, both satisfied and not, to let you see how others rate the site.

The Difference Between Homeopathic HCG and HCG Injections

Homeopathic HCG is created from the full-strength, synthetic HCG hormone used for injections. The homeopathic version is diluted and made into sublingual drops that can be placed under the tongue, usually three to six times per day.

The amount of the homeopathic HCG hormone in your system is taken in a continuous flow to reap the same benefits you would have with the injections. The homeopathic HCG version is easier to use and less intimidating than the HCG injections. It's also a less expensive route to take if you've decided that you want to try the HCG hormone and diet plan.

The homeopathic HCG hormone version is used in conjunction with the HCG diet plan and takes from 20 to 40 days to complete, depending on how much weight you want to lose. The weight loss plan also consists of a low calorie diet during which you only ingest 500 calories per day.

One good thing about the HCG diet plan is that there is no thinking about which foods you can eat during the 500 calorie phase. Dr. Simeon, the researcher who introduced the weight loss plan back in the 1950s, is very specific about the combination of foods you should eat during the low calorie diet phase.

Some enthusiasts for homeopathic HCG, claim that the HCG hormone took away hunger and cravings during the diet and that they never gained the weight back. The reason for these claims could be that the HCG hormone taken during the weight loss diet is designed to reset the hypothalamus so that it's functioning at normal levels.

If you've dieted off and on for years or have taken antibiotics, your hypothalamus may not be operating at its optimum level. The hypothalamus gland is in charge of calibrating the metabolism so that it's burning fat calories and stored body fat at a rapid rate for weight loss.

The HCG weight loss program is a "holistic' plan that teaches your mind and body how to be emotionally and physically fit and many have said that going through the homeopathic HCG plan has given them a new lease on life. People simply feel better when they have a new body image combined with the natural effects that the HCG hormone provides.

Choosing homeopathic HCG over HCG injections is a wise choice for many who find that going to a doctor to get the injections is expensive and time consuming and that giving the injections to yourself could cause bruising and soreness if you're not properly trained on how to give them. Taking the oral drops is simple and produces the same results.

Homeopathic HCG doesn't have to be refrigerated because it's formulated using a small amount of alcohol. The alcohol preserves the integrity of the HCG hormone and keeps it active and effective.

The homeopathic HCG oral drops combined with the HCG diet plan has helped thousands lose unwanted weight and keep it off. They're available online and at some homeopathic pharmacies.

The Difference Between Homeopathic HCG and HCG Injections

The HCG Plan Includes Hormones and Diet

You may have recently heard of the HCG plan and are wondering what it's all about and if it could be the answer to your weight loss problems. The HCG plan has been the answer for thousands of others – and it could be just what you're looking for.

The HCG plan consists of a strict and regimented diet, plus injections or sublingual oral drops of a synthetically-produced HCG hormone. The oral drops have recently been developed and introduced because injections were so intimidating for most people.

Kevin Trudeau launched the version of the HCG plan that caught the attention of people who had tried every diet plan known to man only to regain the weight (plus more) after they stopped the diet. Trudeau maintains that it's ridiculous to think that people can stick to a diet plan that offers pre-packaged food that tastes like cardboard or a lifetime of few and tasteless calories.

Trudeau's book, "The Weight Loss Cure," highlights the late Dr. A.T.W. Simeon's research back in the 1950s which led to the discovery that the HCG hormone can trigger the hypothalamus gland and restart sluggish metabolisms that are so necessary to weight loss and to keeping it off. Combined with a strict, 500-calorie diet plan for a few weeks, the weight loss is fast – and permanent.

The HCG hormone is naturally produced in the placenta of a pregnant woman to ensure that the fetus and the mother receive nutrients necessary to a healthy pregnancy. Now, the hormone can be produced in its synthetic form and given to both men and women in the form of injections or oral drops.

There are three phases to the HCG plan. The first phase is a cleansing process, where the body is prepared for the other two phases to come. Phase one also includes a couple of days of binging on foods high in calories and fats – creams, avocados and cheeses and foods high in carbohydrates are part of the process. The reasons for this binging protocol is to jump start the body into the pattern of burning extra fat calories.

Now, your body is prepared for Phase 2 of the HCG plan. Phase 2 includes taking injections or oral drops of the HCG hormone and can last for as long as 40 days, depending on how much weight you have to lose. This phase is the extremely low calorie – 500 – part and what you can eat is carefully explained in Dr. Simeon's, "Pounds and Inches," which is downloadable at various sites on the Internet.

Trudeau also explains the diet in his book, "The Weight Loss Cure," and innovative recipes for the HCG plan are abundant on the Internet. With the use of seasonings and herbs and some creativity, most of the meals can be made more interesting.

Phase 3 of the HCG plan is the maintenance phase of the diet, where the food choices are much better than during the previous phase. Most people don't regain the weight – most likely because their metabolisms have been reset and they've adapted to better eating habits.

What You Should Know About HCG Phases

The HCG weight loss diet plan isn't like any other diet you've ever tried. It isn't a fly-by-night plan that's going to make you purchase aids such as pre-packaged food or special equipment for exercising. This diet only requires that you put your body and mind through certain HCG phases designed for optimum results.

If you follow the HCG phases explicitly, you'll reap rewards and benefits that you never thought possible. The HCG plan is based on a diet that is combined with HCG synthetic hormone injections or sublingual drops. As you're approaching a decision to try the diet, keep in mind that you should plan to complete all the HCG phases for the best outcome and long term effects.

In the first phase of the HCG diet plan, you'll be going through a detoxifying process designed to get your body – and your mind – ready for what's to come. You'll be drinking lots of water and eating very few calories.

Second of the HCG phases is the most fun part. You'll binge on calories – eating the foods you've been dreaming about during the first phase. But, this phase only lasts for a couple of days. This phase probably sounds like the strangest one, but it's specifically designed to reset your metabolism and ready your body for the third phase.

The third phase is when you begin taking HCG hormone injections or sublingual drops. As you progress, your hunger pains and cravings will subside and you'll notice that your body is actually beginning to reshape itself.

After the third phase, the pounds you wanted to lose are a distant memory and you're ready for the final HCG phase. The maintenance phase of the HCG diet plan guarantees that you'll maintain your new and ideal weight, even though you've reached the end of the HCG doses.

This HCG technology was perfected by the late, Dr. A.T.W. Simeon over thirty years ago, but made popular with the controversial book by Kevin Trudeau, "The Weight Loss Cure." In his book, Trudeau chronicles his weight loss journey with the HCG hormone injections and even inserts photos of the process.

Trudeau also explains the theory behind the "cure," which involves the HCG (human Chorionic Gonadotropin) hormone that's originally produced by cells in the placenta of a pregnant woman. Now that the hormone is synthetically produced, it can be used in this highly effective weight loss plan in the form of injections or drops inserted beneath the tongue.

The diet plan and HCG phases have evolved and been perfected since Dr. Simeon's research back in the 1950s. It's now recommended that you take supplements during the dieting phase, when you're only consuming 500 calories per day.

After religiously following all HCG phases, people have testified that the results for weight loss have been absolutely amazing and that they have a new lease on life because they don't expect to put the pounds back on.

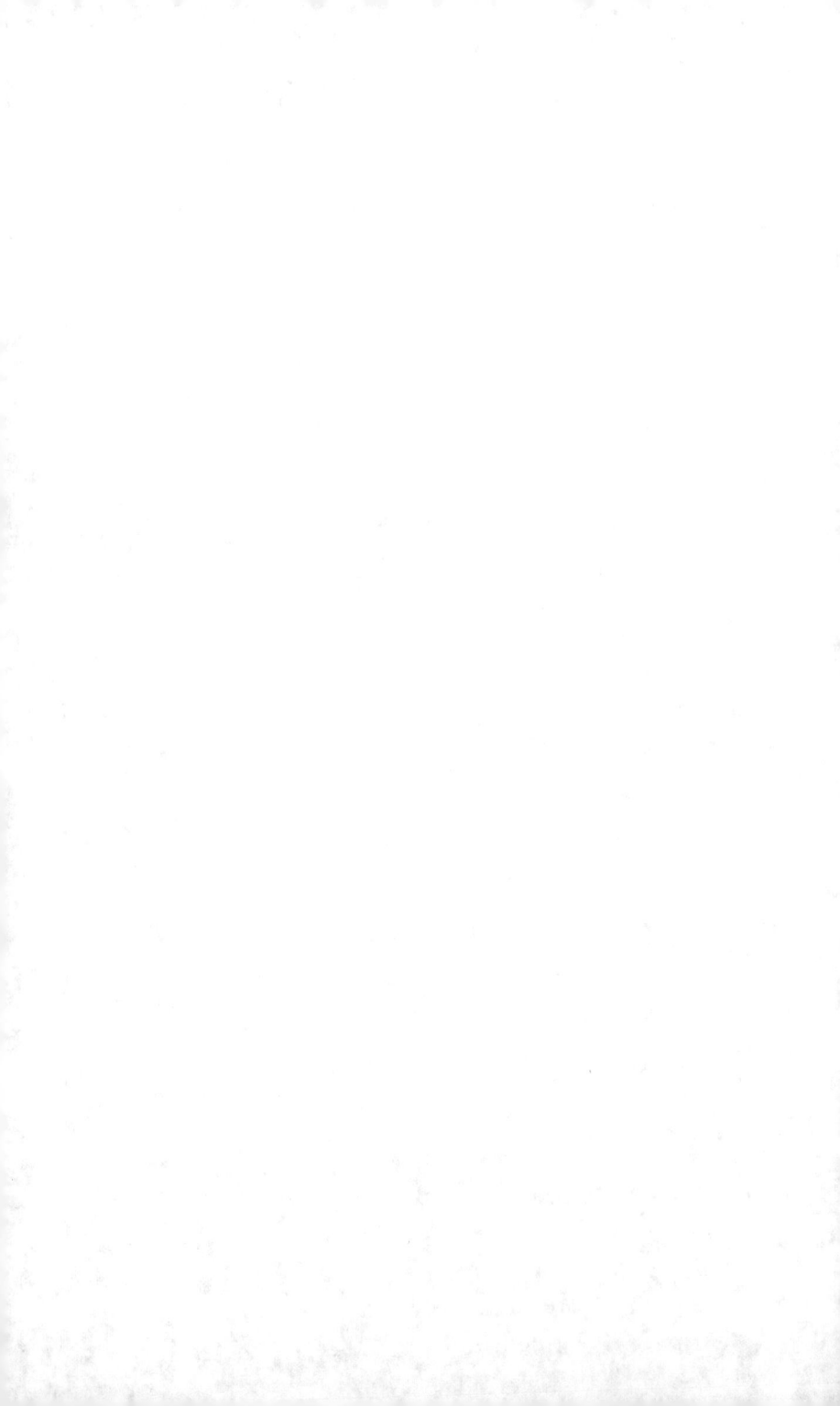

What You Should Know About HCG Side Effects

Any diet program can cause some side effects if your body is even mildly shocked from eating new and different types of food, ingesting fewer calories or beginning a strenuous exercise program. There may be fewer HCG side effects with this diet plan than most others because it's composed of three phases designed to ease your system into the plan.

If you've researched the HCG diet plan at all, you know that its ultimate success depends on the synthetic human gonadotropin hormone. The actual hormone is produced by pregnant women and forms the foundation of a healthy pregnancy. The synthetic version was first offered in injection form, but side effects of pain, bruising and soreness was a deterrent to staying on the plan.

Now, the HCG hormone is offered in oral drops which can be safely and easily used by men and women to help lose unwanted pounds and return both body and mind to a healthy state of being. Thousands who have benefited from the weight loss results achieved by the HCG diet plan have reported that the outcome far surpassed any uncomfortable side effects.

Although HCG side effects are rare, some do occur on occasion if your body reacts negatively to the use of the HCG hormone. Most of these reactions subside within a few days. Some side effects that have been reported include headaches, especially at the beginning of the treatments. This side effect can happen in many diet plans that involve the release of toxins from the body.

Tiredness and mental fatigue can have also been reported as HCG side effects. This can occur when the HCG hormone triggers fat to move to the bloodstream so that it can be circulated and released from the system. This type of HCG side effect usually happens during the first part of the plan when the metabolism is adjusting to the change.

Other complaints associated with HCG side effects have included dry skin and leg cramps. It's easy to understand this side effect – there's such a small amount of fat being consumed that your body can easily become dehydrated. This complaint can be eradicated by taking supplements or some simple medications prescribed by your doctor.

Some women may worry about HCG side effects in regards to future fertility issues. Unlike other, newer diet plans, the HCG diet has been effective for many years and thousands of women have had successful results – and no side effects that could affect fertility. In fact, the HCG hormone is sometimes used to promote fertility in women.

Because the HCG diet plan includes a phase that is extremely low calorie – 500 calories per day for a certain amount of time – exercise should be monitored carefully. If you begin or continue with an exercise program that your body isn't accustomed to, you could run the risk of burning more calories than are available and starving yourself.

Again, most HCG side effects have been associated with the injections and not the oral drops, so if you're concerned about side effects of the plan, consider using the drops. They've been proven to be just as effective as the injections.

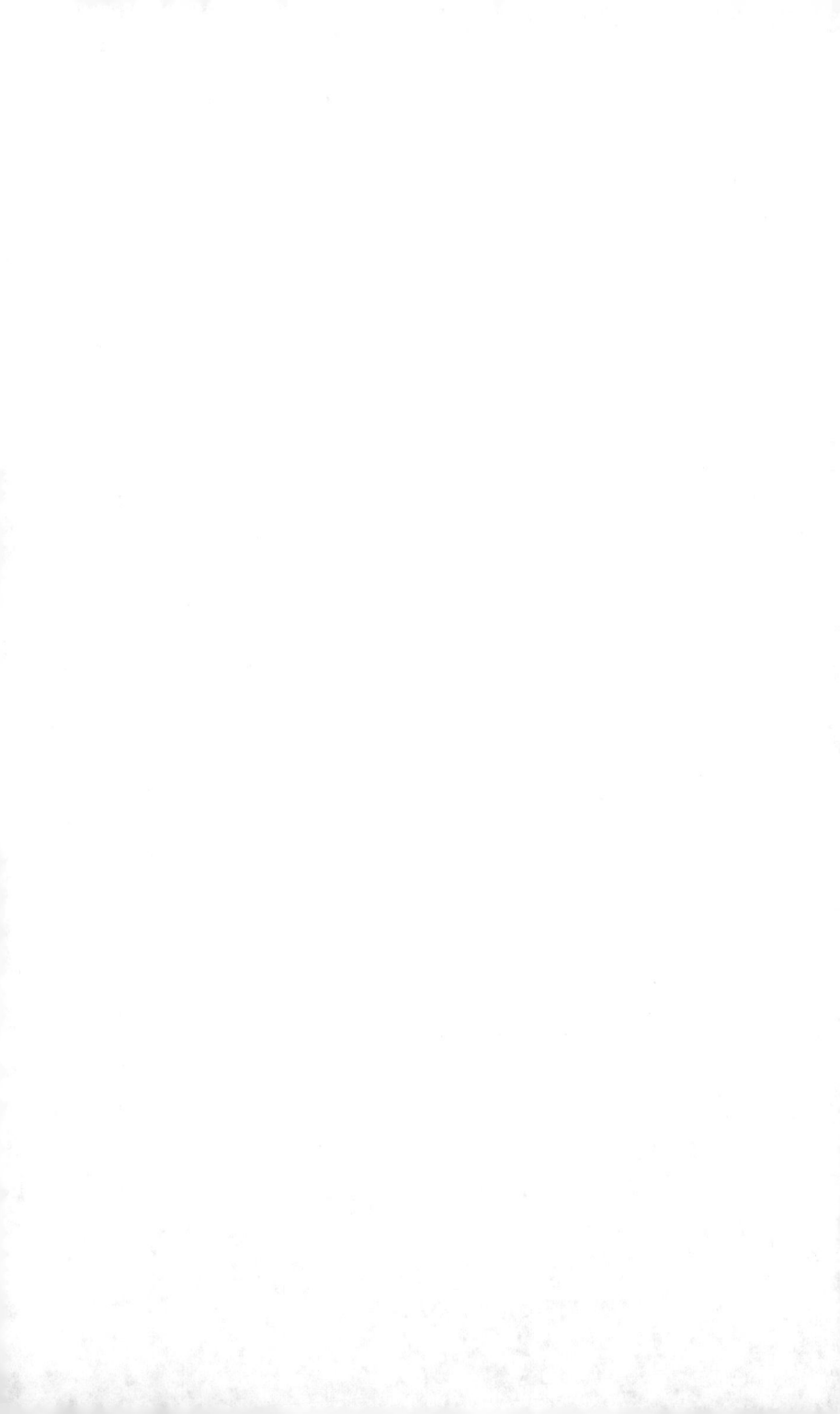

Where You Can Find the Best HCG Diet Recipes

The HCG diet plan is becoming well known to millions who are searching for a plan that really works. As a result of this newfound popularity, HCG diet recipes that ease the restrictive 500 calorie per day phase now abound -- both online and in books that you can purchase almost anywhere.

When the late Dr. Simeon began researching the HCG diet plan more than 30 years ago, he issued a protocol for all of his weight loss patients that they had to adhere to if the plan was to work. It's a simple diet designed to minimize calories while fueling your body with what it needs to interact and be most effective when used with the HCG hormone drops or injections.

Simeon was very specific about portions and types of food involved in his diet plan. Partakers of today's HCG diet plan can find free, new and improved HCG recipes by accessing online sites such as Facebook and official HCG diet sites.

If you prefer enhancing the HCG diet recipes with fresh or packaged seasonings or adding new twists to dishes that can taste boring, there are gourmet sites and cookbooks available. Most offer free, downloadable recipes and information that can help you along as you progress through the three phases of the plan.

Let's face it, when food is more interesting to prepare and ingest, the diet can be much more successful in achieving long term effects. Sometimes that's a bit tough with the HCG diet, since the approved list of foods is so short. That's why it's important that you incorporate interesting recipes into the diet plan that have been formulated from reputable HCG homeopaths or distributors.

There are definitely ways that you can be creative enough with the HCG diet plan so that you're not constantly bored with the choices. For example, one free online site offers a method to bring more variety into the list of foods you must stick to. Apples can be sliced and dusted with cinnamon or cut into cubes and microwaved with cinnamon, cardamom and a bit of clove.

Finding unique and interesting recipes is an extremely important part of the HCG diet plan. If you become bored with this restrictive diet, you may fall off the wagon, and that would be a shame if you've invested money in the HCG hormone drops or injections and spent time researching the plan.

Many HCG dieters who have tried the plan before you have used innovative methods to add interest to the recipes without compromising the integrity of the diet plan. Some of these dieters have started blogs or web sites that you can easily log on to and take advantage of their tips and solutions.

HCG diet recipes will help you rethink what you know about eating healthy foods. As you become innovative with your own recipes, you'll begin to realize what triggers hunger and food cravings and which foods and seasonings can satisfy your cravings and help you continue with this life-changing diet plan.

An HCG Chart Can Help You Plot Your Weight Loss Progress

With any diet plan, you need to see how your weight loss is progressing – has it leveled off at times or revved up at other times? An HCG chart will help you plot your progress when you embark on the HCG hormone and weight loss plan.

Online guides that explain how you can lose weight by following the HCG plan are available both to purchase and to download free. Of course, the guides and information that you purchase may have more data you can use, but the free downloadable guides work just as well most of the time.

It's important that you keep track of exactly how your weight loss is affected as you follow the path of injections or oral drops of the HCG hormone. The HCG chart might also have room for remarks. There, you can jot down what you've eaten and the caloric intake for the day, week and month.

Promoter of the HCG weight loss program, Kevin Trudeau, used a journal and chart to plot his remarkable progress on the diet and hormones. The late, Dr. Simeon, creator of the HCG diet plan also charted the weight loss of his patients over 30 years ago when he was conducting research.

Simeon's patients' weight loss was amazing, but it wasn't until Trudeau came across the charts and information the late doctor had chronicled that the weight loss plan became known to millions. The HCG weight loss plan was very controversial at the time Trudeau released Simeon's findings because the FDA hadn't approved the synthetic hormone.

At that time, the hormone had to be given by doctors by injection or in the form of a prescription for the shots. Today, the synthetic hormone has been approved and formulated into oral drops that anyone can purchase and insert under the tongue to receive the same benefits as the injections.

Online information on the HCG diet plan is abundant now. You can read how others kept an HCG chart and how it helped them stick to the diet and reap the benefits. You can also purchase other supplies from the online sites such as pre-packaged salad dressings and other seasonings and food that help you with portion size.

Supplements are also available to enhance the HCG diet plan and ensures that you're getting the nutrients you need while going through the low-calorie diet phase of the plan. Trudeau suggests that you prepare your body for the HCG hormone and diet by a cleansing technique, and you can also find information for that procedure online.

Keeping an HCG chart can be a mental catalyst for you to continue on the HCG hormone and diet plan. It's easy to forget how much you've progressed and what you did to get there, so glancing at a meticulously kept chart can help you realize what worked and what didn't and give you a mental boost to keep on going.

Confused About HCG Diet Phases?

The HCG diet plan is becoming increasingly popular as stellar results are reported, but there is some confusion about the HCG diet phases because of conflicting information available on the Internet. Some of that information contradicts itself. The confusion is usually associated with the difference between the late Dr. Simeon's HCG plan and Kevin Trudeau's plan.

Both men tout the HCG weight loss plan, but the HCG phases they recommend are a bit different. Each plan works, and you should gather all the information you can before you begin. You might notice after your research that Trudeau recommends that cleansing should occur within Phase 1 of the plan and before you take in a large amount of calories.

Phase 1 of the original (Simeon) plan doesn't include system cleansing. Simeon's plan calls for you to "load up" on calories, eating cheeses, cream sauces, avocados and other fat-laden foods. The theory of the caloric increase in Phase 1 is that your body will be alerted to the fact that an over-abundance of fat calories are being ingested – and need to be burned off.

During Phase 2 of the HCG diet phases, you'll begin what is arguably the most important part of the HCG diet plan. You'll begin to take HCG hormone injections or sublingual drops every day for 20 to 40 days, depending on how much weight you want to lose. Phase 2 also includes an extremely low calorie diet. Each day you're on Phase 2, you'll eat no more than 500 calories.

This amount of calories per day may seem that it wouldn't sustain a normal person who's performing normal, calorie-burning activities. But, working together with the HCG hormones you'll be taking, this HCG phase delivers everything it promises. Even though you're not ingesting a lot of calories, your hypothalamus gland is busy working to stimulate your metabolism so that you're burning stored fat calories – and this is what leads to weight loss.

Your hypothalamus gland may have become sluggish and non-active from years of yo yo dieting and other factors. The HCG hormone acts to stimulate the gland so that it does its work much more efficiently and actually resets your metabolism. That's why people who have gone through the HCG phases report that the weight doesn't reappear after they stop taking the hormones and go back to a normal diet. The metabolism keeps on working.

Phase 3 of the HCG diet plan is the maintenance phase. This phase lasts for three weeks before you reenter phase 1 again and go through the "loading on calories" phase. If you go around again, you'll add another week onto Phase 3. How many rounds you choose to be on the HCG diet plan depends on the amount of weight you want/need to lose.

One round of HCG phases might be all you need, but if you fit into the obese category, it may take as many as three or four rounds before you lose all the weight. Also, on the second round, the diet restrictions are significantly less, meaning that you can add more foods and ingest more calories than when you were on the first round.

Confused About HCG Diet Phases?

It's important that you stick to the plan of the three HCG phases. Any deviation from the original plan might mean that you don't reap as many rewards – or lose as much weight.

Following the HCG Protocol

The HCG protocol for losing weight is like no other diet plan you've ever followed. The difference in this diet plan and the others is that this one really works. You'll be amazed at how the pounds melt off your body – and it's been around for over thirty years.

An HCG protocol involves using either HCG shots or liquid drops inserted beneath the tongue. Following the diet plan and the hormone regime will reset your metabolism so that it keeps burning fat calories even when the diet ends. It doesn't matter which method you decide to use – they're both equal in their effectiveness for weight loss.

Along with HCG hormone injections or oral drops, you'll complete three diet phases designed to jump start your metabolism. HCG followers say that the hormone they're taking during the extremely restrictive diet quashes their hunger pains and cravings, making it much easier to stick to the 500 calorie per day regimen.

If you decide to adhere to Dr. Simeon's HCG protocol, you'll choose the injections over the drops and the HCG diet plan will be much more restrictive. Kevin Trudeau, who wrote the controversial book about HCG, entitled, "The Weight Loss Cure They Don't Want You to Know About," suggests adding vitamin supplements to the regimen and bring interest to bland foods by using spices.

Either HCG protocol is said to produce the same results, and most people are reluctant to give themselves injections, so the oral drops would be the best choice. As for the HCG diet plan that accompanies the injections or drops, Trudeau's method of spicing up the flavor of the meat, vegetables and fruit will help you stick to the diet plan and not become bored with its limited offerings.

You may also choose to get HCG injections is from your doctor, but that's an expensive solution to the HCG protocol. A doctor could also give you a prescription for the shots or you could order them from an online vendor. Just be sure you're getting the real thing and that the company you're ordering them from is reputable.

One factor in the HCG protocol for weight loss is that no or very little exercise is recommended or required. During the 500-calorie per day diet, your body will become weak from the shock of so few calories to keep it going, so on those days you should rest and conserve your energy.

HCG diet fans have said that after awhile they regain their energy levels and even have more than they're accustomed to. Other side effects that some HCG protocol followers say they've experienced are headaches, irritability, tender muscles, bloating and water retention. These side effects aren't experienced by most people and tend to go away after a few days.

The HCG protocol isn't always easy to follow, but if you want a fast, reliable weight loss plan that will reset your metabolism and burn fat calories even after you stop the plan, the HCG diet plan may be what you're looking for.

Get Free HCG Information Online

If you're thinking about trying the popular HCG diet plan, you should know that there is free HCG information available online. You can download most of the information you'll need to give you a head start in knowing what's involved in this remarkable new weight loss breakthrough.

The HCG diet plan includes a period of time when you're eating extremely low calorie (500) meals. Since the recommended foods can sometimes be bland and tiring, it's important that you spice them up with various seasonings and try new recipes that won't compromise the results of taking the HCG hormone.

Part of the free HCG information that's available to you online are recipes, seasonings and other methods designed to make the food more palatable. This is especially helpful if you've got a great deal of weight to lose and you're going to be on the diet for more than a month.

Free HCG diet plan information might also include data about others who have experienced the diet plan and what results they've had. There are blogs that you can join and chat or exchange information with others about how you're progressing once you begin the HCG hormone and weight loss plan.

There are three phases of the HCG weight loss plan and tons of free HCG information online about each one and what you can expect during each phase. It's important that you understand what's going on inside your body and mind and how to cope with weakness, headaches and other feelings that may occur during each phase.

Before you decide if you want to use the HCG injections or the easier to use oral drops, you should access the free HCG information online that details the methods and the side effects of each one. You'll also find out which method you think would suit your needs and best fit your lifestyle.

When you're thinking of starting on any diet or exercise program, you need to get all the information you possible can before you force your body to accept foreign drugs or foods you're not accustomed to eating. Free HCG information on the Internet can give you peace of mind as you research the plan and before you decide it's the right one for you.

After you begin the HCG hormone and diet plan, you may have questions about how you're feeling or what's happening to your body. You'll be able to find loads of information that you can print out or download for your convenience.

Free HCG information is definitely a good way to research the HCG hormone and diet plan. Just be sure the information is from a reputable site and that coincides with what professionals say about how the plan can help you lose the weight you need to lose and keep it off for the rest of your life.

HCG Phase 3 Sets Up Your Metabolic System

After Phase 1 and 2 of the HCG diet plan, Phase 3 seems relatively simple. You begin HCG Phase 3 on the day immediately following the last day of Phase 2. Phase 2 was the extremely restrictive part of the plan, where you took HCG injections or sublingual drops. Now, you'll be allowed to eat any type of food you desire – and as much as you want. But, there are some exceptions.

Foods that are prohibited during HCG Phase 3 are:

· Sugar, honey, molasses, dextrose, sucrose, high fructose corn syrup or sweeteners.
· Starches, including pastas, all wheat products, breads, potatoes, rice, yams, etc.
· Artificial sweeteners
· Fast foods
· Foods containing nitrates
· Cold drinks
· Foods containing hydrogenated or partially hydrogenated oil and trans fats.

You should also avoid constant air-conditioning, florescent lights, drink lots of water, take a walk each day, eat organically grown grapefruit and apples, take a teaspoon of raw coconut oil two times per day, drink organic teas, eat a large breakfast and several snacks per day. Don't go to bed until 3 to 4 hours after you've eaten your last meal and get plenty of sleep.

Staying calm and stress free is also an important part of HCG Phase 3. Take deep Yoga-style breaths several times per day and meditate if you can. Avoid television and listen to calming music. You may want to take vitamin supplements during this phase.

Be sure to weigh yourself every morning after urinating. This is an important part of charting your weight loss and discovering if what you're doing each day is working positively toward your ultimate goals.

Your weight should begin to stabilize during HCG Phase 3, and your metabolism will adjust itself so that it keeps burning unwanted fat calories. Your weight should remain within two pounds of the weight you registered on the last day you gave yourself an HCG injection or took the sublingual oral drops (during Phase 2).

If the scale suddenly shows that you've gained two pounds, you should fast until 6:00 pm that day. During that time, you'll drink as much water as you can – one gallon at the most and half a gallon at the least. You may also drink some of the recommended HCG teas, using stevia to sweeten it. At the end of the day, you can have an organic grass fed beef steak and a large tomato or apple.

After completing HCG Phase 3 of the HCG weight loss plan, you should feel highly energetic and happy. You'll no longer be slave to the cravings and binging that were part of your life before HCG.

HCG Reviews – The Good And the Bad

Once in awhile a diet plan comes along that gets fantastic raves and reviews. Then, it slithers out of sight because it runs the gauntlet of people who have tried it – and failed. HCG reviews keep coming in – some bad, but mostly very good.

We spend thousands of dollars on diet plans that sound so easy to follow. Pre-packaged foods delivered right to our door are the current craze. It looks delicious in magazines and on television, but when we actually do the "taste test," it falls way below our level of tolerance.

The HCG (human Chorionic Gonadotropin) hormone and diet plan has been around for over thirty years. It works because it speeds up our sluggish metabolisms and rids your body of unwanted fat cells that are burned off at a higher rate of efficiency.

Some HCG reviews claim that the 500 calorie per day diet plan would make anyone lose some weight – and that's true. But, as soon as normal food intake occurred, the weight would reappear along with a few more pounds. The HCG diet plan is different because the hormones taken during the low calorie diet phase work to reset the metabolism by stimulating the hypothalamus gland, ensuring that those fat calories will continue to be burned off.

HCG reviews that claim the diet plan didn't work can be very misleading. Delving deeper into the reasons why the plan didn't work usually reveals that these reviewers didn't follow the plan explicitly.

Dr. Simeon, the founder of the HCG plan and Kevin Trudeau, who wrote the book, "The Weight Loss Cure They Don't Want You to Know About," implicitly state that the diet won't work unless you adhere to the plan they outline in their books.

HCG reviews are often simply complaints about the strictness of the diet and the blandness of the recommended food. Trudeau took the HCG diet plan a bit further by recommending that certain seasonings be used to make the food more interesting, and now, you can purchase salad dressings and seasonings to help make the bland food more palatable.

Other HCG reviews claim that headaches occur along with irritability and light-headedness. This is true about almost any other diet that restricts caloric intake. It's a fact that your body will react in different ways when you're beginning any type of lifestyle change. Exercise and diet plans often bring negative results, but almost always – it's temporary.

After your body becomes used to the diet and hormonal changes, you'll feel better than you ever have before. Most reviews from those who have been faithful to the HCG diet plan have reported that they never regained the lost weight and had more energy than ever.

You can read online HCG reviews at many online blog posts and HCG sites and make your own decision about whether the good outweighs the bad with this weight loss plan.

How Can an HCG Shot Help Me Lose Weight?

The HCG (human Chorionic Gonadotropin) hormone is commonly used to stimulate ovulation in women who ovulate so infrequently that it's almost impossible to become pregnant. When a woman receives an HCG shot, the ovaries are stimulated to produce eggs and then release them. If an HCG shot is given to a man, he'll have help in producing testosterone at a normal level.

When an obese person is given one shot of HCG hormone per day for 20 or more days, it acts to stimulate the hypothalamus gland, which may be inactive and a main cause for obesity. The stimulated hypothalamus gland then stirs up a sluggish metabolism and causes the body to lose unwanted fat and leave lean muscle mass intact.

The late Dr. A.T.W. Simeon researched the HCG shot's effect for weight loss in the 1950s, but it wasn't really popular until Kevin Trudeau recently publicized the method and results of Simeon's research. Some of the studies included Indian women and overweight boys who were given HCG shots to stimulate fertility in women and puberty in boys.

Both the women and the boys lost weight when they took a daily HCG shot in conjunction with a very low calorie diet plan. After further research, it was determined that HCG shots changed the way in which the metabolism functions, speeding it up to burn unwanted fat calories that are responsible for obesity.

For those who have struggled with obesity all their lives, getting one HCG shot per day is a piece of cake compared to the pounds that have made their lives miserable all those years. Now that HCG injection "kits" are available, some people are giving themselves an HCG shot rather than paying more to have a doctor administer it.

If you're intimidated or afraid of giving yourself a shot, there is now another method to get the full benefits of the HCG hormone. A synthetic HCG hormone has been developed and can now be purchased in oral drop form that's inserted sublingually. The HCG shot is only taken once per day, whereas the drops must be taken two or three times per day, depending on the strength of the formula.

The diet plan that accompanies the HCG shot is very restrictive. You're only allowed 500 calories per day while you're getting HCG injections or taking the oral drops. There is much information online about the diet plan and various ways you can enhance the flavor of rather bland foods.

During this diet phase of the HCG diet plan, your metabolism will be stimulated by the HCG hormones in your body and will burn stored fat, rather than recently ingested fat calories. This serves to reset the metabolism so that it keeps working even after you stop the diet and hormone therapy.

One HCG shot per day over a 20 day period can help you lose the unwanted pounds you've been trying to get rid of for years. Do your own research to find out if this plan might work for you.

How Do HCG Diet Plans Differ from Others?

The main difference between HCG diet plans and other weight loss plans is the fact that you also take regular doses of the HCG hormone as you're dieting. The HCG hormone comes in two different forms – oral drops and injections.

The HCG diet plans also include a strict limitation of caloric intake. When taking the injections or drops and limiting your calories to 500 calories per day for a certain amount of time (depending on how much weight you want to lose), the system is burning at least 2,000 calories simply from the stored fat in your body.

While other calorie-based diets usually suggest certain food groups to choose from, HCG diet plans require that what you eat is from a highly specific menu. For example, when the menu calls for chicken breast, you shouldn't substitute turkey breast.

There are certain seasonings that you can use liberally on plain foods to make it more palatable and interesting. Seasonings such as cinnamon and cardamom can be sprinkled on fruit such as apples. These types of seasoning don't add calories and are acceptable to use on HCG diet plans.

The HCG hormone that's included in HCG diet plans serves the purpose of stimulating the hypothalamus gland. When this gland is stimulated, your metabolism is recalibrated and works at burning fat in a rapid and efficient manner even after you stop taking the HCG hormones.

HCG diet plans require that you go through three phases of dieting. Phase 1 is a low calorie phase and might include cleansing of the body system. This can proceed for several days. At the end of the low calorie part of the first phase, you'll binge on high calorie foods.

This phase is important and much different than most diet plans. You might think of the end of this phase like a car that's run out of gasoline. It begins to sputter, trying to use every last drop of gas to run on. As soon as you fill up the car with more gas, the engine begins to run smoothly.

Your body is working the same way on HCG diet plans. During the low calorie phase, your body is using fat that's been stored in your body to get every ounce of energy it cans to keep the body running. During the binging process, the body resets itself and the metabolism that's designed to burn fat begins to purr and do its job efficiently.

Kevin Trudeau made HCG diet plans popular with the publication of his book, "The Weight Loss Cure They Don't Want You to Know About." Trudeau's book is based on the findings of the late Dr. Simeon who researched HCG diet plans and the effect that the HCG hormone had to reducing fat in obese people.

Trudeau's theory was that the FDA didn't want the news to get out about the HCG hormone and HCG diet plans because it would make other diet plans defunct and millions of dollars would be lost by companies who base their profits on diet plans that don't really work.

How to Know If You're Getting the Correct HCG Dosage for Weight Loss

HCG dosage for weight loss should be carefully monitored to be sure you're getting the correct amount of the hormone for your size and weight. The HCG hormone is available for men and women in the forms of pills, oral drops and muscle injections, and those over 16 years of age can take from 125 to 200 i.u. each day.

Taking too much of an HCG dosage might result in muscular cramps, headaches, nausea and vomiting, so be sure you're getting the correct HCG dosage. But, HCG for weight loss has been shown to really work if you want to lose those stubborn, unwanted pounds. In combination with the diet plan, an HCG dosage will stimulate the hypothalamus gland – which in turn, revs up your metabolism.

Before you purchase the HCG hormone in any form, be sure you know what the true strength is. Some drops have an additional amount of alcohol or water, diluting the recommended HCG dosage, so be sure you know what each HCG dosage contains or the plan may not work as well for you.

Some followers of the HCG weight loss plan have reported losing 20 to 40 pounds in a couple of weeks, and have also noticed a marked improvement in bulges and flabby muscles. HCG is a glycoprotein chemical that breaks down fats from all parts of your body and turns them into energy before flushing them out of the system.

Essentially, you're on a 500 calorie per day diet while you're taking the HCG dosage, but the hormone serves to trick the system into thinking you're taking in more calories because the metabolism keeps working to burn the calories that you've stored into fat cells.

The jump start to the metabolism takes place after you've ingested a high amount of calories for a couple of days. You'll eat such foods as avocados, cream sauces and other high fat and calorie foods. When you begin the strict diet along with the HCG dosage, your body will still be burning those fat cells, but this time it will burn the ones you've stored rather than the ones you've ingested.

There are three ways you can take an HCG dosage – pills, drops and injections. The pills and oral drops are taken 2 to 4 times per day, depending on the amount of weight you need to lose and the strength of the pills and drops you purchase.

If you're taking the HCG injection route, you'll probably only need one shot per day because injections normally come in higher HCG dosage. Whichever way you choose to take the HCG hormone therapy, you shouldn't exceed more than 200 i.u. per day.

Exceeding the proper HCG dosage might result in headaches, muscle cramps and light-headedness. If you experience these side effects, rethink the HCG dosage you're taking.

Learn All About the Weight Loss Plan on An HCG Forum

As the HCG weight loss plan has become more popular, information in the form of HCG forums have popped up all over the Internet. If you want first person accounts of what others know about the HCG weight loss plan and how successful it's proved for others, an HCG forum is definitely where to look.

You'll find everything you need to know about the HCG weight loss plan, including opinions about the debate over whether to take HCG injections, pills or sublingual oral drops for the best results. You can also find out the best and least expensive online sites from which to purchase HCG products.

People exchange recipes on HCG forums that will help you discover better ways to prepare the food. During the diet phase of the HCG weight loss plan, your calories will be limited to 500 per day. And, the foods that you must eat have to be the exact ones listed on the plan. Most of the foods are boring and bland unless you perk it up by following a tried and true recipe.

Some HCG forums include journaling from those who have tried the HCG weight loss plan -- and you can learn a lot from these – especially if you're a newbie to the plan. The highs and lows that others experienced while on the plan can tell you volumes about where the problem areas will be and help as you take your own weight loss journey.

On one HCG forum, you can find varied results from followers of the plan. One person may be posting about the fabulous results he or she experienced while another might say that she never lost weight, but gained some on the plan. There are such a diverse collection of comments and reactions to HCG that you'll need to follow along carefully to see which you believe.

Helpful information that you can find on an HCG forum includes what to do after getting off the plan. Now that you've lost all the weight you needed to lose, what's next. On an HCG forum you'll see the methods that others are using to keep it off.

The subject of using teas and supplements on the HCG diet plan enjoy lively discussions on HCG forums. Certain types of teas are recommended by actual partakers of the diet and you can also find recommendations about supplements to take during the diet part of the plan and how others were affected.

HCG forums have a respected place in online information sites. Years ago, we'd never have had the camaraderie that's offered today simply by joining or following a forum that's discussing subjects we're interested in. If a problem keeps reappearing or a certain product gets bad reviews in an HCG forum, it's a good idea to check it out before you try the same thing.

Keep in mind that the information you see on an HCG forum may or may not be correct – and some suggestions might not work for you and what you're looking for.

Low Calories Make Up Allowed HCG Foods

The original HCG diet plan, formulated by the late Dr. Simeon, was made up of HCG foods that are extremely low in calories. Foods such as veal, beef, chicken breast fish, some crustaceans, vegetables such as spinach, beet-greens, tomatoes and cabbage and simple fruits such as strawberries or grapefruits.

Since the HCG diet at its lowest calorie point is only 500 calories per day, HCG foods consist of what will fill up the dieter and provide the most strength to get through the low calorie days. You can also have tea or coffee in any quantity, but only one tablespoon of milk is allowed within a 24 hour period – and Saccharin or Stevia may be used as a sugar substitute.

In Kevin Trudeau's book, "The Weight Loss Cure They Don't Want You to Know About," the HCG foods change a bit and seasonings are more liberally used. There are also recipes for HCG foods in abundance on the Internet. Cookbooks also now exist and the recipes don't stray far from the ones that Dr. Simeon used, but they're more interesting to eat.

There are even pre-cooked and packaged HCG foods that you can purchase online, such as HCG diet approved vinaigrette salad dressing, garlic breadsticks and Cajun seasoning to spice up a boring piece of meat. Some HCG foods come in "packs" that you can buy all at once and contain much of what you'll need to spice up HCG meals.

Although Dr. Simeon didn't recommend diet supplements in his original HCG diet plan, "Pounds and Inches," Kevin Trudeau does recommend them in his "Weight Loss Cure" book. Some diet supplements that are recommended to enhance diet results are Homeopathic Cell Salts and Homeopathic Vitamin B-12.

It's your choice whether you want to follow the original, "pure" plan of Dr. Simeon or the enhanced plan of Trudeau. You may want to read what's included in each man's diet guidelines and decide for yourself which plan is right for you. If you don't have a lot of weight to lose, the original plan might not be so boring that you're tempted to stray from it since you won't be on the diet as long.

There are all types of guides and cookbooks available for purchase, online or in your favorite book store. There are also sites on the Internet that let you download as much information as you need to begin and see you through all the theories and HCG foods you'll need while you're on the diet.

As the HCG diet has become super popular, some companies are offering HCG foods that are perfectly proportioned, meats that are defatted and fast-frozen. They come to you in the mail, so all you have to do is pop them in the freezer and warm them in the microwave when you're ready.

Scams are out there, so be sure you research the authenticity of the HCG foods that you purchase and that they follow the guidelines set forth by Simeon or Trudeau.

The Phenomenon of HCG Diet Drops

HCG diet drops have become the new weight loss phenomenon in today's world where everyone is trying to lose those nagging pounds they can't seem to get rid of no matter which diet they choose or which exercise program they adopt.

The strange caveat about this diet phenomenon is that hGC (human Chorionic Gonadotropin) has been around for years. It's naturally produced in pregnant women to enhance the development of the fetus. Back in the 1950s, Dr. A.T.W. Simeons began to do research with obese women and boys and found that the HCG hormone actually stimulates the hypothalamus gland, which regulates the metabolism and keeps rein on triggers such as cravings that cause us to overeat.

We're all born with HCG hormone levels, but as we go through life, chemicals in the food we eat and other diet factors cause the levels to decrease until finally, we're left with inactive cells that contain the hormone. This situation does us no good at all when we're trying to lose weight.

HCG hormone injections worked to increase HCG levels, but had to be administered by a doctor – and this was an expensive process. Many doctors also knew little about the diet plan that must accompany the injections to be successful. As a result, these injections were seldom used on patients to help them lose weight.

The HCG hormone and diet plan came to prominence after Kevin Trudeau, a controversial consumer activist, began his own research based on the findings of Dr. Simeons, and lost a ton of weight on the plan. People were clamoring for the HCG hormone, but didn't want to give themselves injections or go the expensive route of having it done by a doctor.

A synthetic form of the HCG hormone was developed, which made way for the creation of HCG diet drops. These drops can be placed sublingually under the tongue and provides the same benefits as the injections.

The HCG diet drops are less expensive, safe and easy to use -- and their effectiveness in shedding pounds from your body has been proven time and again. If you follow Simeons' weight loss plan, you'll pair the HCG diet drops with the strict diet that he recommends.

Simeons' HCG diet plan consists of a variety of healthy foods from all food groups. You're only allowed 500 calories during a certain amount of time during the plan, but you're taking the HCG diet drops at the same time, so most of your hunger and cravings are curtailed.

Weight Loss Using HCG, Dr. Simeons Protocol

Dr. Simeons never saw the popularity of his HCG hormone research reach the heights that it is today. Dr. Simeons began research using HCG for weight loss in the 1950s and wrote a manuscript entitled, "Pounds and Inches." Documenting the protocol for HCG, Dr. Simeons' research revealed astounding results after administering the hormone to obese Indian women and boys.

After some time of giving injections to the women and boys involved in the experiment, Dr. Simeons noted that significant amounts of weight were lost and the bodies of these people began to reshape naturally, without exercise or any effort on their parts.

Continuing with treatments of HCG, Dr. Simeons noted that weight maintenance after the injections were stopped, didn't present a problem. The weight stayed off and the metabolism continued to burn fat calories at an effective rate.

This amazing weight loss breakthrough didn't become popular right away. Most people are intimidated by giving or getting daily injections, and going to a doctor to get the shots was expensive. But, when a synthetic HCG hormone was developed, the diet plan and HCG dosages became plausible.

When Kevin Trudeau, the controversial consumer advocate, became enamored with HCG, Dr. Simeons' research came to light and Trudeau tried the weight loss plan using Dr. Simeons' protocol for himself. Trudeau found ways to tweak the diet so that it became easier to accomplish in today's world of pre-packaged foods and over-the-top diet plans.

Trudeau's protocol includes a cleansing procedure at the beginning of Phase 1, but Dr. Simeons' original protocol didn't call for that measure. Both protocols call for a couple of days of high caloric and fat intake, followed by an extremely low calorie diet plan – only 500 calories per day.

Both Trudeau and Dr. Simeons are specific about which foods you should eat on the diet phase of the weight loss plan. Trudeau found some ways to improve on the flavor of some of the bland offerings without compromising the calories or the nutrients of the foods.

With today's protocol of HCG, Dr. Simeons would possibly be shocked and delighted that now there are pre-packaged HCG diet foods, measured to the exact proportions and recommended calorie count and shipped right to your home. There are also salad dressings and seasonings you can purchase that will greatly enhance the flavor the food.

In further research of HCG, Dr. Simeons also reported in his manuscript that obesity was a problem that would continue and threaten our health as a population if a remedy wasn't found.

What Is HCG – And Can It Help Me Lose Weight?

The question, what is HCG, can be answered with the technical definition that it's a hormone (human Chorionic Gonadotropin) that's produced in the cells of the placenta of pregnant women. It helps the fetus and the mother enjoy a healthy pregnancy by providing much needed nutrients to both.

Everyone, including men, has the HCG hormone in their bodies, but it resides in cells that are normally not active. The synthetic form of the hormone is now being used along with a diet plan to help people lose weight and keep it off.

The synthetic HCG hormone, when taken by injections or oral drops, triggers the hypothalamus gland to break down and use body fat as the main fuel source for the body. That's the reason for the extremely low (500) calorie diet that accompanies the intake of the HCG hormone.

When your body isn't receiving a large amount of fat calories for the hypothalamus gland to break down, it begins using stored fat cells. Another purpose of the gland is to send a message to the brain aimed at conserving and keeping lean muscle. If your body was not receiving this message, you'd begin to reduce important muscle mass.

So, the answer to the question, what is HCG, includes the fact that without the hormone injections or oral drops and sticking to the HCG diet plan, you wouldn't realize the same results as most people who adhere to the plan religiously.

Basically, the HCG hormone is fooling the body into thinking it's getting the calories it must have by replacing the ingested calories with stored fat calories that are keeping you overweight and miserable.

The HCG diet plan lasts about 20 days and provides an ocean of benefits to your body and mind. Now, you'll diet and restore the energy you seem to have lost over time. Now, you'll be able to fit into the "skinny" clothes hanging in the closet. Both your body and mind will enjoy a transformation that could only take place if your metabolic balance is fixed.

All the weight loss plans in the world won't work if your metabolism stays sluggish. After you get off the diet, the weight will automatically fly back on. HCG ends this vicious cycle by providing long lasting results that will reset your slow metabolism and keep the weight off permanently.

You'll also fall into new eating and exercising habits that will keep your body fit and lean. The HCG hormone and diet plan isn't a magical cure, but it's a cure that does what it claims and makes you a happier and more fulfilled person because you'll become that fit person you always knew you could be.

Think of the answer to what is HCG as a fabulous new "discovery" that ends the roller coaster ride of losing and gaining unwanted pounds. Check it out yourself and see your health care provider before you begin any weight loss plan.

When It Comes to HCG, Phoenix, AZ Leads the Way

Weight loss clinics have popped up all over Phoenix, Arizona, and most offer information and injections or sublingual drops of HCG. For spa retreats and HCG, Phoenix offers many programs for weight loss, but the HCG weight loss program is by far the most popular with people who have tried and failed to lose weight in the past.

These spas and clinics offer specialized weight loss doctors who treat men and women on a daily basis and have had remarkable successes. Most are very affordable, and if you're intimidated by giving yourself injections of HCG, Phoenix clinics might be an option to consider.

The HCG diet was developed and researched by Dr. Simeons in the 1950s, but made popular by controversial consumer activist, Kevin Trudeau. Phoenix, Arizona was one of the first areas to jump on the bandwagon of this increasingly popular weight loss plan and as a result, clinics and spas have sprouted up all over Phoenix offering HCG injections and guidance for the plan.

HCG is a hormone that's produced naturally by the placenta in a pregnant woman to help develop the fetus into a healthy and strong baby. Now, there's a synthetic version of the hormone that can be given to men and women to help them lose unwanted pounds.

Within clinics and spas that specialize in weight loss and HCG, Phoenix is a leader. Many also offer personal trainers to help promote further muscle toning and therapy so you'll receive the maximum benefits from HCG. The HCG hormone injections or oral drops are accompanied by a rigorous diet plan that restricts your caloric intake for a period of time.

Sometimes, the diet plan can be confusing. Specified portions are recommended and the food on the diet can be bland and uninteresting unless you know how to spice it up. Only 500 calories are allowed during a portion of time while you're on the diet, and it can become tiring if you don't know how to make it more palatable.

When people began to become aware of HCG, Phoenix spas and clinics immediately recognized that this was a plan that worked. The HCG hormone works in conjunctions with the diet to reset your metabolism by stimulating the hypothalamus gland. That's why people who choose this weight loss plan rarely put back on the weight they lost. The metabolism keeps on functioning effectively to burn off unwanted fat calories.

When the hypothalamus gland isn't working properly, you'll have food cravings, hunger and imbalances that leave you weak no matter how much or how well you eat. Then, as the hypothalamus gland is stimulated by the HCG hormones, it begins to work effectively to burn fat calories.

If you're thinking of going to a spa or clinic to receive HCG, Phoenix can provide many for you to choose from. Most of these clinics are designed to give you all the help and guidance you need to lose those undesired pounds.

About the Creator Of the HCG Diet, Simeons

If you ventured onto a site for an amazing new weight loss plan called HCG, you may want to know more about the creator of the HCG diet, Simeons. The late, Dr. A.T.W. Simeons is credited with performing experiments on reducing obesity during the 1950s.

Simeons viewed the problem of obesity as a jig saw puzzle waiting to be put together. Some parts of the cure involved solving the impulse to overeat, some involved the person's body system and others had to do with inactive or sluggish parts of the body that could help get rid of unwanted fat cells if they only worked properly.

Natural remedies were inexpensive and used in other countries, but unknown in America. Dr. Simeons knew that if he could prove that a natural remedy could help cure the problem of obesity, that it could change lives everywhere – including America.

While developing his theory about curing obesity and the HCG diet, Simeons used the HCG hormone in injection form to administer to his patients who needed to lose weight. Simeons' theory was that the HCG hormone, produced by the placenta in pregnant women to bring nutrients to the fetus, could also be used to stimulate the hypothalamus gland and reset the metabolism.

Used along with the HCG diet Simeons developed, the plan would ensure that a person's metabolism would keep burning fat calories even after the diet and hormones were finished. This plan was a non-surgical and natural method that would help people lose unwanted pounds and embark on a life style they had always dreamed of.

Simeons' HCG hormone and diet plan was highly successful during the experiments he conducted on overweight Indian women and boys. His manuscript, "Pounds and Inches," produced scientific evidence that the HCG protocol worked to melt pounds and inches from people suffering from obesity.

Amazingly, it wasn't until consumer advocate, Kevin Trudeau, came across these scientific findings did the HCG diet, Simeons' version, become popular. Trudeau chronicled his own weight loss of forty pounds and dubbed the breakthrough as, "the weight loss plan they don't want you to know about."

A synthetic form of the HCG hormone was developed and people who suffered from weight loss clamored for this new "cure." In fact, it's become so popular that HCG diet recipes, seasonings for the rather bland diet and tips and hints to aid in the success of the plan have popped up all over the Internet and homeopathic health pharmacies.

Search the Internet if you want to know more about the HCG diet, Simeons' protocol and how this weight loss plan can help you lose those unwanted pounds now and forever.

Choose an HCG Clinic – Or DIY?

As the popularity of the HCG weight loss plan increases, so are HCG clinics. If you do a google search for an HCG clinic, you may find one in your own city. If you don't, it's simply a matter of time before one appears. In fact, they're popping up faster than google can keep track of them, so check in your local directory before you give up.

Why go to an HCG clinic? HCG clinics offer supervised weight loss using the HCG protocol developed by the late Dr. A.T.W. Simeons. Most clinics offer injections or use of the synthetic form of the HCG hormone in oral drops. At an HCG clinic you should receive personalized supervision that tracks your weight and diet plan and can alert you if there are problems involving your health.

The HCG weight loss plan involves injections, pills or the oral drops of the HCG hormone while following a highly restrictive (500 calorie) diet plan. You can purchase injection "kits" online, but, unless you know how to give injections, you might suffer from bruising and pain that can be avoided if administered from a professional. You can easily take the HCG pills or insert the oral drops sublingually, but you may need guidance about the dosage you should take.

The main advantage to seeking out an HCG clinic is the supervision aspect. You should receive counseling from beginning to end of the weight loss plan. A highly professional staff should also provide diet education and consultation sessions that will keep you on target for the weight you need to lose.

As with any weight loss plan, supervision is preferred over going it alone. But, if you see your regular physician and he or she pronounces you fit for the plan, you may want to proceed on your own. You can purchase injections, pills or oral drops online and go for the DIY route, or opt for the HCG clinic. Either way, you should be carefully monitored for the duration of the diet and taking the HCG hormone.

Most HCG clinics follow Dr. Simeons' HCG diet plan protocol, but may also offer hints and tips about how to make the diet's bland food more interesting. They'll also offer recipes or tell you how to purchase pre-packaged foods if you hate shopping for and putting together the recipes yourself.

You may be the type of personality that has to have guidance for your weight loss journey or it may not work. A plethora of guidance books, HCG forums and blogs and just about anything else you would need to go it alone exists on the Internet, but if you can and are willing to pay for the extra attention you'd receive at a clinic, it might be worthwhile.

Just as there are online scams about everything on the Internet, there may be fly-by-night HCG clinics that are here today and gone tomorrow. That means you should carefully research the credentials of the HCG clinic before paying a fee or entrusting your weight loss goals and overall health.

Finding An HCG Calculator for Weight Loss

When taking the HCG hormone and using the HCG diet plan to lose unwanted weight, an HCG calculator can be used to measure your BMI (Body Mass Index). An HCG calculator can also be any calculator that helps you with weight and portions of food. These calculators are often used for obesity-related health problems and diseases such as hypertension, diabetes and heart conditions.

If you're using an HCG calculator to measure BMI, you want to be sure that your BMI is below 25 at all times. When you measure BMI, you're using your height and weight to determine the calculation. Sometimes BMI overestimates the body fat in persons, and this usually occurs when the person is very muscular people.

An HCG calculator is typically used to measure Beta HCG levels in pregnancy. HCG levels usually increase by doubling every two days during the first four weeks of pregnancy and as it progresses, it slows down considerably. An HCG calculator can be used by entering the date of a blood test and the beta HCG level for that day. Enter the beta HCG level for the following blood test and you can then calculate the progression of the HCG hormone.

If you're trying to lose weight, you can also use a caloric intake calculator as an HCG calculator to determine how many calories have been burned during the HCG diet plan. One pound of fat equals 3500 calories per day, so if you're on the

500 calorie per day HCG diet, the results should roughly be one pound per week.

Most of the time our bodies don't work as efficiently as the calculator predicts, so you should take into consideration other elements involved during the HCG weight loss plan. As the HCG hormone stimulates the hypothalamus gland and your metabolism improves, the weight should begin to melt off rapidly, since you're burning calories more efficiently.

Another useful HCG calculator that can be used in the weight loss plan is the nutrient calculator which breaks down your current diet into protein, fat and carbs. A "bulking calculator can be used to measure weight or muscle gain.

It's been proven that our bodies react to lower calorie levels by reaching a "weight loss plateau," which tends to be discouraging if you're still torturing yourself with an extremely low calorie diet.

The only way to truly counteract this weight loss plateau is to increase the metabolism, which is exactly what the HCG hormone diet plan has been proven to accomplish. Use the many weight loss calculators on the market as an HCG diet calculator to determine how rapidly you're losing weight on this remarkable weight loss plan.

HCG Diet Reviews Reveal Pros and Cons

You can find out a great deal about the HCG weight loss plan by reading online HCG diet reviews. Since HCG is a controversial weight loss method, you should know the pros and cons before starting on this unique weight loss journey.

HCG stands for "human Chorionic Gonadotropin," and is a special hormone that's produced naturally in the placenta of a pregnant woman. The synthetic version of the HCG hormone, when administered by injections, pills or oral drops, is part of a weight loss program that has become extremely popular. It serves to stimulate the hypothalamus gland which in turn resets your metabolism.

The HCG weight loss plan includes a diet that's highly restrictive, using only 500 calories per day. Online HCG diet reviews include the pros and cons of embarking on such a drastic weight loss plan, and data about others who have tried the plan and been successful – or failed.

There seems to be no middle-of-the-road position in whether or not the HCG diet plan works. HCG diet reviews that are for the plan tout the immediate results achieved when you follow the course as outlined by the late Dr. Simeons. Simeons was the man who researched the HCG hormone when used for weight loss and carefully outlined a specific course to follow to achieve maximum results.

Most of the HCG diet reviews that are against the plan say that HCG hormone injections can cause pain and bruising. Luckily, there are oral drops and pills that can be taken as an alternative. These online sites also claim that the low caloric diet can cause light-headedness, irritability and headaches. But, that's true for any low calorie diet plan.

HCG diet reviews can also be helpful when choosing a specific product. Since online scams exist, you should have recommendations about which sites offer pure HCG products and which could be diluted or possibly even dangerous to take. These products might also discourage you from following the diet plan if no results are achieved.

Any confusion about the diet portion of the HCG weight loss plan can be alleviated by finding HCG diet reviews that offer more details about the plan and some offer recipes and tips for achieving ultimate success.

There are HCG diet reviews that point out possible dangers in using the HCG hormone in conjunction with the HCG diet plan. Even though the HCG hormone is approved by the FDA for fertility treatments, it isn't approved by the FDA as a weight loss treatment. Despite that fact, HCG seems to cause no harm to individuals as long as you're taking the recommended dosage.

If you're worried about using the HCG weight loss plan to achieve your weight loss goals, by all means take advantage of the HCG diet reviews that offer information about the pros and cons before making a decision.

HCG Shots for Weight Loss – Safe or Dangerous?

HCG (human Chorionic Gonadotropin) injections are typically used to treat infertility in women by stimulating ovulation or increasing sperm count in men. HCG shots for weight loss is a fairly new plan that came to light when Kevin Trudeau, controversial consumer advocate, came across Dr. Simeons' research on using the hormone for a weight loss cure and popularized the plan.

Although the FDA hasn't approved HCG for weight loss, it's been approved for fertility, so the synthetic version of the hormone can be sold – either online or in homeopathic health product stores. As of today, manufacturers of the synthetic HCG product for weight loss must state on the product that no substantial evidence for weight loss suggests that HCG shots for weight loss are effective.

There are instances in which a person considering HCG shots for weight loss should beware of. For example, if you don't know the proper protocol for giving yourself injections, you should consider taking pills or oral drops – or going to a doctor or HCG clinic to have them administered.

Otherwise, you might suffer from a number of maladies, including abdominal swelling, nausea, vomiting or diarrhea. Even though online HCG injection kits explain the proper procedure, it's sometimes intimidating to give yourself an injection. If you have concerns, you should seek help from a professional before using HCG shots for weight loss.

Blood clots may also occur if you don't know the procedure for HCG injections. Also, you may experience a rash, hives, swelling around the mouth or breathing difficulties. These are rare side effects if you're taking HCG injections for weight loss, but you should know about them just in case.

Another con for taking HCG injections for weight loss is that pregnant women or women who may become pregnant can run the risk of a multiple pregnancy. If you're using HCG injections for weight loss, you should stop taking the hormone immediately if you become pregnant.

The evidence for using HCG injections for weight loss is clear when you research the subject online. There's an abundance of people who post amazing results on the HCG hormone and diet plan and most say they've never regained the weight because their metabolism was reset and now works efficiently to burn off unwanted fat calories.

If you're considering using HCG injections for weight loss, you should also be aware that unless you purchase the product from a reputable online site or homeopathic pharmacy, you run the risk of being stuck with a faulty product and one that's not going to deliver the results it promises – or that you hoped for.

If HCG shots for weight loss are prepared and delivered correctly, they should be effective and safe. If the thought of getting injections scares or intimidates you, consider using the HCG oral drops or pills to achieve your ultimate weight loss goals.

Planning Your HCG Menu

You've decided to go for the HCG weight loss plan to lose those unwanted pounds finally and forever. That means you're now faced with planning an HCG menu that you can stick to while taking HCG hormone injections, oral drops or pills.

The HCG menu plan according to Dr. Simeons' protocol for rapid and permanent weight loss is restrictive, utilizing only 500 calories per day while you're taking the HCG hormone. Following the menu plan is critical for the success of the diet, so planning the HCG menu is one of the most important tasks you must perform.

An HCG menu may be restrictive, but if you have enthusiasm and determination for this weight loss plan, your attitude can help you over the hurdles and get you to your ideal weight. Keep thinking that the radical part of the diet only lasts for 21 days – then, you'll be primed and ready to enjoy your weight loss success for the rest of your life.

Fortunately, there are many guides and help-sites online that can get you through the menu planning and any other questions or concerns you may have about the HCG weight loss plan. Online sites are a good way to familiarize yourself with the HCG menu plan, so be sure and take advantage of all they offer.

According to the prescribed HCG menu protocol, you should eat as much fat-laden food as possible during the first 1 to 3 days of the diet. This includes avocados, cream sauces and desserts with high fat content. This is the fun part of the diet and sets up your metabolism for what's to follow.

The next part of Phase 1 of the HCG weight loss plan includes daily dosages of the HCG hormone which can be accomplished by using injections, oral drops or pills. This portion of your menu plan will include a drastic drop in calories and you'll be restricted to certain foods from specific food groups.

A typical HCG menu plan for breakfast might include 1 egg, plus 3 egg whites either boiled, poached or raw. Tea or coffee is acceptable, but without sugar (you can use Saccarin or Stevia) and only 1 tablespoon of milk. Lunch might include 100 grams of veal, beef, chicken breast, white fish, lobster, crab or shrimp. If you're a vegetarian, you can substitute meat with skimmed milk or cottage cheese in the advised amounts.

Drinking a minimum of two liters of liquid per day is essential and vegetables for each meal should be eaten alone and not in combination with others. Variation is the key to planning a successful HCG menu that will lead to all the rewards you'll receive on the HCG weight loss plan.

Read Online Reviews of HCG Diet to Get the Facts!

Online reviews of the HCG weight loss plan can provide facts you might need before proceeding with the HCG diet. You might also pick up some HCG diet fiction in a review – so it's best that you thoroughly research this controversial weight loss plan before making a decision about whether or not it's right for you.

The HCG diet is used with the HCG hormone in injections, oral drops or pills to achieve weight loss and keep it off. Most online reviews of HCG diet include the fact that the hormone stimulates the hypothalamus gland which in turn resets the metabolism so that you're burning ingested fat calories more rapidly and efficiently.

You can learn a lot from reading reviews of HCG diet, and you can take advantage of some of the review sites that offer recipes, tips and hints about how to follow the plan for lasting success. The HCG diet plan contains very strict guidelines that you must follow for ultimate triumph over obesity.

During Phase 1 – the diet portion of the plan, you'll only be ingesting 500 carefully planned calories per day along with the HCG hormone in shot, oral drops or pill form. Your body will be burning fat cells at a rate of between 2,000 and 3,500 calories per day while you're only putting 500 calories into it.

The results of this restrictive plan is that you might lose anywhere from 1 to 3 pounds per day. The total amount of weight you can lose depends on the amount of time you choose to stay on the HCG weight loss plan. Online reviews of HCG diets can tell you more about how this diet phenomenon takes place and how effective it can be.

You may come across some online reviews of HCG diet that are critical of the plan, but read on and you may find why the plan wasn't effective for this particular reviewer. Most followers who aren't successful usually can't stick to the diet plan over the recommended period of time and some didn't take the recommended dosage of the HCG hormone.

Keep in mind that some online reviews of HCG diet plan are slanted to discourage you because the reviewer offers another weight loss plan that he or she wants you to choose over the HCG plan. But, certain reviews that offer facts can be extremely helpful in the final decision you make a about whether or not the plan is the right one for you.

Kevin Trudeau, the consumer advocate that lost a ton of weight on the HCG weight loss plan, calls it, "the weight loss plan they don't want to tell you about." People who have achieved amazing results on the plan say that hunger and cravings were almost non-existent and that they kept the weight off even after they got off the plan.

Read reviews of HCG diet for yourself and then make your own decision. As with all other weight loss plans, you should see a physician to be sure it's a healthy one for you.

Sublingual HCG – A Fast and Powerful Weight Loss Solution

Sublingual HCG is a fast and effective method of achieving weight loss – and keeping it off. It's much easier than the injection form of the HCG supplement and has proven to be just as potent. Sublingual HCG is much safer than injections too. Going to the doctor to have injections administered can be expensive and time-consuming, and giving them to yourself can be dangerous.

Dr. Simeons, the creator of the HCG hormone injections and diet plan specifically designed to reduce obesity, gave his patients HCG injections during the 1950s and had amazing results that he chronicled in "Pounds and Inches," a medical manuscript.

The HCG hormone is produced naturally by the cells in the placenta of pregnant women and serves the purpose of ensuring a healthy newborn baby. After Simeons' research and success came to light a few years ago, a synthetic form of the HCG hormone was created and people began to follow Simeons' weight loss plan by taking HCG drops sublingually.

Performing injections on yourself might be dangerous if you don't know the proper protocol, but there's very little chance of contamination and other medical problems when you use HCG sublingual drops under the tongue to be absorbed by the mucus membranes.

Studies about sublingual HCG have indicated that it is absorbed into the body at about the same rate as injections and faster than the HCG pill form. And, hardly anyone wants to face an injection every single day for 21 days, even if a doctor is administering them.

The sublingual HCG serum is quickly absorbed into the bloodstream by the multitudes of blood vessels that lie just beneath the tongue. These HCG drops will stimulate the hypothalamus gland, which will regulate your metabolism so that you burn fat calories at a faster and more efficient rate.

The oral pill form of the HCG hormone is effective, but doesn't contain the chemical makeup to absorb into the skin like the sublingual drops. Pills are directed into your stomach, where the enzymes and acids contained there obliterate the effectiveness of the HCG hormone.

You can purchase both the HCG injection kits and sublingual HCG from many Internet sites, but be sure you're getting a pure product and one from a company that's reliable and that manufactures the product in the United States. The U.S.A. has tighter and better control over the way homeopathic substances are produced, so don't risk going out of the country simply because it's cheaper.

Suppliers of sublingual HCG can be found online or in homeopathic pharmacies and are much less expensive than purchasing the injection form of the hormone. Although you may need to take sublingual HCG two or more times a day to receive the recommended dosage, and you'd only need one injection to get the same effectiveness, it's usually much less intimidating to opt for the sublingual drops than shots.

What You Should Know About Side Effects Of the HCG Diet

Most diets have side effects that you should know about – especially if you have a health condition that may prohibit you from trying certain diet plans. If you're thinking of trying the HCG weight loss plan, you should know about the side effects of the HCG diet and problems that may occur.

People who have successfully lost weight on the HCG diet have reported very few side effects – and the ones that did occur could happen in almost any low calorie diet plan that you might undertake. Headaches, light-headedness, irritability and light water retention are sometimes experienced during the diet phase of the weight loss treatment.

Other side effects of the HCG diet might occur if you've opted for injections rather than the oral drops or pill form of the hormone. If you're giving yourself the HCG injections and don't know the proper procedure, you could develop redness and swelling around the injection site.

If you don't know how to properly give yourself an injection, it's best to either let the doctor provide them or select the HCG oral drops or pills instead. A very rare side effect of taking the HCG hormone is called ovarian hyper-stimulation syndrome (OHSS). This usually occurs during the first round of the HCG weight loss protocol and could cause swelling, pelvic and stomach pain and shortness of breath.

Call your health care provider if you experience any of the above side effects. Usually, the HCG hormone and weight loss treatment is all about good side effects. Followers of the HCG diet have reported that headaches, irritability or other common side effects of the HCG diet went away after a few days and that they felt less hunger or cravings than they thought would occur.

The truth is that side effects of the HCG diet plan are usually much less than the risk of obesity it's used to treat. Many successful followers of the weight loss plan have reported that migraine headaches have subsided. Diabetes patients stated that their blood sugars stabilized and others have been awed at feelings of increased energy.

HCG causes an important and fantastic side effect of resetting the hypothalamus gland, which in turn speeds up the metabolism process so that you can burn unwanted fat calories more rapidly and efficiently. A newfound confidence also occurs when you've lost the weight that's kept you from joining in life's most enjoyable activities.

Your self-esteem reaches new highs when you shed the weight and you feel and look better than you ever have before. Some people have reported that the HCG hormone and diet treatment left them with a glow and tautness of the skin that they had never before experienced.

Weigh the pros and cons of side effects of the HCG diet and decide for yourself if this may be a plan you want to know more about. Information on the Internet about the HCG hormone and diet plan can be obtained by a click of the mouse.

What You Should Know About Side Effects Of the HCG Diet

You Can Find Information About HCG Online

Now that the HCG hormone and diet plan popularity has reached a fever pitch you can find information about – and purchase – HCG online. The HCG hormone is now produced synthetically and comes in the form of injections, pills and oral drops. Taking the HCG hormone along with a very restrictive diet has helped thousands lose unwanted pounds.

Tons of information and web sites that offer the product in any form you choose can be found online, and you can even chat with others who are either on the HCG plan, have been on it or are thinking about it. Join these conversations to find out what HCG is all about.

Perform a simple google search for HCG and you'll reap all types of sites, from everywhere in the world. It's a lot of HCG online information to digest, and some are myths while others declare the truth about this phenomenal diet plan that's sweeping the Internet.

Which should you believe and how do you know if the HCG online information is correct? It takes some time researching the subject and carefully choosing the sites to really get the scoop on the HCG hormone and diet plan. There are some tips about getting the correct information.

First, be sure that the Internet site is reputable. Follow blogs, Twitter, Facebook and any other social networking site that contains a thread about the HCG hormone and diet plan.

See what others are saying about the site and the product. You'll eventually notice a pattern about the HCG information you're discovering.

When you're ready to purchase HCG online, be sure that the product is made in the United States. Some foreign countries are producing the product, but the guidelines on added ingredients are sometimes more lax and you may end up not getting what you bargained for.

Also, read the reviews from others who have purchased HCG products from the site. Did they receive it in a timely manner? Were they allowed to use credit or debit cards rather than the Western Union method? If an online site specifies that you must use Western Union to pay for the HCG product, consider it a red flag that the site may be a scam.

You can also find online information about the late Dr. Simeons and how he researched and developed this amazing weight loss plan during the 1950s and how it came to light only recently when Kevin Trudeau, the controversial consumer advocate used it himself to lose 40 pounds.

HCG online information of all types and both pro and con can be used to help you make a decision about whether or not this diet plan is right for you. Just make sure you're getting correct information and that the product(s) you purchase are top notch. Then, you can proceed with confidence.

Index

www.ingramcontent.com/pod-product-compliance
Lightning Source LLC
Chambersburg PA
CBHW062035280526
45788CB00003B/1011